21 USES OF HYDROGEN PEROXIDE

Healthy Uses For A Health Home And Surroundings

Dr. Mike Peters

Table of Contents

CHAPTER ONE

BASICS OF HYDROGEN PEROXIDE

Hydrogen peroxide is different from water most effective via the addition of one greater oxygen molecule. But that greater molecule turns it into a powerful oxidizer. It's the purpose hydrogen peroxide is this kind of versatile cleanser, and

it's also the purpose you want to apply it cautiously on human beings and pets.

Hydrogen peroxide breaks down fast and easily whilst it comes into touch with air or water, so it's taken into consideration safer than chlorine chemicals.

Hydrogen peroxide kills yeasts, fungi, microorganism, viruses, and mildew spores.

The CDC lists unique concentrations you want and how long you want to allow them t ake a seat to kill different organisms.

CHAPTER TWO

USES OF HYDROGEN PERIOXIDE

In your kitchen

1. Clean your dishwasher to take

away mildew and mildew for your dishwasher, spray the problematic components of your dishwasher wherein moisture can linger lengthy after a cycle is complete — inside the pleats of rubber seals, traps, and crevices of the utensil basket.

2. Scrub your sink

I suggest this trick to smooth your kitchen sink: Wet the floor of your sink, then scrub it with baking soda sprinkled onto a sponge. When you've scrubbed the entire surface, pour 3 percent hydrogen peroxide over the surface and permit it to sit earlier than rinsing it smooth.

3. Disinfect counters and slicing boards.

cleansing counters with undiluted hydrogen peroxide is effective at killing E. Coli and Salmonella microorganism on har d surfaces like counters while it's allowed to sit on the floor for 10 minutes at room temperature. A 10-minute soak in 3 percentage hydrogen peroxide to kill germs on timber slicing boards.

4. Wash veggies – and amplify their shelf life. use 1/four cup of 3 percentage hydrogen peroxide consistent with gallon of water to help get rid of bacteria from vegetables. If you're washing delicate-skinned veggies like lettuces, just soak for 20 minutes after which rinse.

Carrots, potatoes, and different tough-skinned veggies may be soaked 30 minutes earlier than rinsing and drying. Because bacteria can motive green s and fruits to turn brown, a hydrogen peroxide bathtub is believed to maintain them clean lo nger for your fridge.

5. Scour cookware. If your cookie sheets, pots, and pans have a baked-on layer of brown, sprinkling them with baking soda, then spritzing the soda with 3 percent hydrogen peroxide will repair them. Allow them to soak for 1 to a

few hours before wiping off the mess.

6. Get rid of rubbish can germs. After washing the garbage can with soap and water, spray the whole box with a 1:1 answer of hydrogen peroxide and water. Let the trash can sun-dry for numerous hours. Just as peroxide cleans surfaces, it'll help dispose of germs from your trash can.

Bathroom uses.

7. Deep smooth your toilet hydrogen peroxide is powerful at removing microorga nisms, which

include microorganism,   yeasts,
fungi, viruses, and spores, making
it a

great choice for cleaning your toile
t.

To smooth your   toilet,   add half
of cup   of   3 percent hydrogen
peroxide to your toilet bowl to kill
germs and brighten the surface of
your   toilet.   You'll need to
leave it within   the bowl   for
20 mins to get the total benefit.

8. Glass   and   shinny   surfaces.
Spray   a   1:1 solution of   and
hydrogen peroxide and water into
glass   surfaces,   then   wipe   with
paper   towels,   a   lint-

unfastened cloth, or newspapers
for a streak-loose clean.
9. Kill mould and mold.
Mould
and mold can construct up quickly
within
the moist surroundings of a
shower stall.
To kill them while not having to
breathe in poisonous bleach
fumes, spray with undiluted
3 percentage hydrogen peroxide
and permit it to sit for 30 minutes.
Rinse. The peroxide will kill the
mould and mold, but you
could still need to cast off the
stains they left behind.

10.   Whiten old porcelain

If your porcelain pedestal sink has yellowed, you could brighten it by using scrubbing   the   dampened sink floor with baking soda, then scrubbing with a sponge saturated with 3 percent hydrogen peroxide.

CHAPTER THREE

MORE USES

11. Foam away cleaning soap scum
For weekly cleansing of a fiberglass shower and tub, make a foaming paste from 1 cup baking soda, 1/four cup white vinegar, plus a tablespoon or two of hydrogen peroxide. When the bubbles subside, scrub the floor of the shower with the mixture.

In the laundry room

12.Hydrogen peroxide as an effective way to eliminate grass stains, blood stains, and drink stains like fruit, juice, and wine. Try dabbing the cleanser at the reverse facet of the cloth to start.

13. Brighten dingy whites Nystul also has a answer if your T-shirts, sheets, and towels have taken on a grimy, grey hue. Make your personal oxygen-bleach by way of combining 1/2 cup washing

soda — hint: It's no longer similar to baking soda — and half of cup hydrogen peroxide. Start the cycle, allow the washing machine to fill, and soak the garb for a couple of hours before finishing the cycle to whiten and sanitize.

In the lawn.

14. Germinate healthy seeds. soaking seeds in 1 to three percent hydrogen peroxide can soften the seed coat and start germination. If you want to growth the chances of

a great plant yield, you may soak seeds in hydrogen peroxide for 20 mins before planting.

15. Clear algae out of your pond water.

If you've got a water function or koi pond, you may properly deal with the water to reduce or eliminate harmful alg ae. Gardening professionals at Get Busy Gardening used 1/2 cup of 3 percentage hydrogen peroxide to clear a 90-gallon pond.

16. Treat flowers with fungal infections

If   your lawn vegetables are laid low

with powdery mould or different f ungal   infections, you   may spray them   with   a   hydrogen peroxide solution to rid them of the   fungus.
Mix 4 teaspoons   of   hydrogen peroxide in a pint of water and spray   the   plant.   Stronger concentrations should burn sensiti ve leaves,   so   don't   use   it   at full energy.

For   your   pets Most

veterinarians not advocate the

usage   of hydrogen   peroxide

to easy your puppy's

wounds, regardless of how small the injury is.

17. Induce vomiting for poisoned dogs
If   your pet has eaten something poisonous,   your veterinarian   may suggest you to apply hydrogen peroxide to make the   animal   vomit. Because   hydrogen   peroxide is risky to   your puppy to   ingest, it's crucial that you talk to your vet or a poison manage center earlier than attempting to set off vomiting with   this   method.
18.   Clean   out   the clutter box
To get rid of odors and disinfect

your   cat's clutter box,   empty
the muddle,   wash
the container with cleaning
soap and hot water, after
which spray thoroughly with   full-
strength peroxide.   Let   it take   a
seat for   15 minutes earlier
than rinsing,   drying,
and changing the litter.

NOTE

Some   aquarium   hobbyists   use
hydrogen peroxide to control algae
and smooth their
tanks, but communicate to   a   fish
veterinarian before putting hydrog
en   peroxide for your tank. While
hydrogen   peroxide
degrades rapidly in   water, a

few species
of decorative fish, which
includes gourami   and
suckermouth catfish, can't tolerate
it.
While   it   does   kill micro
organism, it   is   able
to be dangerous to
fibroblasts, which   are cells
your frame needs for   healing.
Don't   lighten   your pores   and
skin with   it
Dermatologists may use hydrogen
peroxide   to deal
with some skin conditions, but it
isn't considered a secure way to
lighten hyperpigmentation in at-
home use.   The risks outweigh

any capacity benefits, mainly due to the fact there are different ways to lighten darkish spots for your skin. Don't use it to treat acne Yes, it bubbles and fizzes and kills micro organism, together with the micro organism which could purpose pimples. But a 2005 examine shows that hydrogen peroxide can also lead to scar formation, so the usage of it directly on acne isn't an awesome concept.

19. Do use it to sanitize your toothbrush and retainer Tiny amounts of those bacteria don't normally caus

e health problems, however in case you need to be on the safe side, soak your toothbrush in hydrogen peroxide.

20.   use it to sterilize make-up brushes   and   kits. After   washing extra make-up off your   brushes   with a gentle shampoo, soak the bristles for 10 mins in a bowl of water with a teaspoon of 3 percent hydrogen peroxide.   You also   can use   it to clean the pads to your eyelash curler. Rinse off any residue very well to shield your eyes.

21.   Do whiten your teeth products are effective and safe wh ile used   properly.__Mix   equal amounts hydrogen peroxide with water, such as 1/2 cup to 1/2 cup. Swish this mixture around your mouth for about 30 seconds to 1 minute. Stop and spit out the solution if it's hurting your mouth and try not to swallow any of the mixture

22.   Do recall letting a professional lighten your   hair Hydrogen   peroxide is commonly considered secure in business hair

dyes, severe chemical burns can happen, even in a expert salon.

Hair dyes with peroxide can harm your hair in case you use them too often, so talk to a educated stylist to exercise session a time
table that'll shield your hair and pores and skin.

CHAPTER FOUR

CONCLUSION

Hydrogen peroxide is a household chemical that may be safely used for a selection of cleansing purposes in your house. Although it was once generally used to disinfect cuts and wounds, it isn't encouraged for that cause today.

Hydrogen peroxide can lessen the likelihood that you'll get sick in case you use it to disinfect surfaces, produce, and other gadgets in your house. Don't apply it to your pores and skin, don't swallow it, and don't try sturdy concentrations of food-grade hydrogen peroxide to try to treatment illness. When used properly, hydrogen peroxide is still a helpful family disinfectant and fitness resource.

THE END

www.ingramcontent.com/pod-product-compliance
Lightning Source LLC
Chambersburg PA
CBHW060850260726
48661CB00002B/724